Natural Eye Care Series:

Dry Eye Syndrome

Supporting Healthy Vision Naturally

Marc Grossman, OD, LAc. and Michael Edson, LAc.

ISBN 9781513663128
Library of Congress Control Number: 2020940765

Printed in the United States of America
Published by Safe Goods
561 Shunpike Rd., Sheffield, MA 01257
SafeGoodsPublishing.com

Natural Eye Care Series: Dry Eye Syndrome is not intended as medical advice. No claims are made for the ability of products mentioned to treat, cure, or prevent any disease. No promise is made for health, and no diagnostic or health claims are stated. This literature is for informational purposes only and is not meant to diagnose, or prescribe for, any health condition. Always see a doctor for matters relating to your health. The FDA has not evaluated this information.

Natural Eye Care: Dry Eye Syndrome

TABLE OF CONTENTS

AUTHORS

Marc Grossman, O.D., L.Ac., co-founder of Natural Eye Care, Incorporated. is best described as a holistic eye doctor. He uses a multi-disciplinary approach using nutrition, eye exercises, Chinese Medicine and lifestyle changes. These provide him with a wide array of tools and approaches to tackle difficult eye problems. Dr. Grossman lectures nationally on natural vision care philosophy and method and teaches workshops for health care professionals including physical therapists, chiropractors and body workers, social workers, occupational therapists, and other optometrists. He is a consultant to school systems, rehabilitation centers and the U.S. Military Academy at West Point. He is co-author of the acclaimed *Natural Eye Care, Your Guide to Healthy Eyes and Healing* (published Jan. 2019), and *Magic Eye Beyond 3D: Improve Your Vision (Volume 6 2004)*, and also *Greater Vision* (2001).

Michael Edson is a co-founder and President of Natural Eye Care, Inc. He is co-author of *Natural Eye Care: A Comprehensive Manual for Practitioners of Oriental Medicine* and *Natural Eye Care: Your Guide to Healthy Vision and Healing*, 2019. Recent titles are *Natural Parkinson's Support: Your Guide to Preventing and Managing Parkinson's* (2020). His upcoming book, *Natural Brain Support: Ways to Help Prevent and Treat Dementia and Alzheimer's Naturally* will be published in 2020.

PREFACE

Natural Eye Care Series: Dry Eye Syndrome offers a unique approach to supporting healthy vision from early childhood to mature age, with the understanding that healthy vision relies on overall health and emotional health. Filled with wisdom and insight of both ancient and modern-day healing methods, this book integrates a wide range of alternative therapies as they apply to health of the surface of the eye.

This book will help you make sensible, researched, and clinically based decisions to support eye health with recommendations that include Western herbs, nutritional supplements, Chinese medicine, and additional therapies. You will learn about the underlying causes and be given tools and techniques to develop your own eye health strategies. If a particular problem, cluster of symptoms, or changes in vision occur, consult your eye doctor.

Natural Eye Care Series: Dry Eye Syndrome shows you how to become an active participant in your own vision care. The primary goal of this book is to offer a practical approach, based on the underlying philosophy that emphasizes prevention and support. In doing so, we celebrate the healing power within all of us and the mind/body's inherent potential for self-healing.

Many eye care professionals give increasingly stronger and stronger prescriptions that help weaken the eyes. Instead they could offer eye exercises and lifestyle recommendations to help strengthen vision. Diet, exercise, lifestyle, and targeted supplements should be a critical part of the discussion of how to maintain healthy vision, even with such eye conditions as cataracts. The peer reviewed research is abundantly available in demonstrating these many alternatives.

This guide is part of an ongoing series educating readers about their vision difficulties, explain prevention strategies, and explore ways to help preserve vision for those with vision disorders. It will enable the individual to be a more informed consumer when it comes to vision care. Medication and surgery may sometimes be necessary or even appropriate treatment strategy, but nutrition and lifestyle choices always play an essential role in helping support healthy vision.

Doctors in China have reached out to the West to borrow the modern medicine we can offer. We in the West can, in turn, benefit from the ancient wisdom of the East. By combining the medical approaches of the East and West, along with other alternative health modalities, we may be able to achieve better health with less cost and greater success in helping patients preserve vision.

Natural Eye Care Series: Dry Eye Syndrome is dedicated to the belief that a common ground can be created in which the strengths of modern Western medicine are united with the preventive approach of other healing modalities.

DRY EYE SYNDROME

Seventy-five percent of those over age 65 experience dryness of eyes, due to a decrease in the production of tears and often due to a tear-drainage dysfunction. The resulting ocular tear-film reduction impacts visual function and comfort, even though it may not directly reduce vision clarity.[1] For men, there is a weak relationship between low androgen levels and dry eye.[2] In the aging population, dry eyes can become a particularly annoying problem, and if it is severe enough and not treated, it can cause damage to the cornea.

The most frequent complaint to eye doctors is dry eyes, known as dry eye syndrome (or dry eye disease), aqueous insufficiency, or meibomian gland dysfunction with consequent reduction of meibum, which protects the tear film from evaporation. Note that retinoids used in cosmetics promote this type of dysfunction.[3] Twenty-five percent of patients who visit ophthalmic clinics report symptoms of dry eye, making it a growing public health problem and one of the most common conditions seen by eye care practitioners.[4] In the United States moderate and/or severe dry eye affects more than 3.2 million of the female population and 1.6 million of male, at or over the age of 50.[5]

TYPES OF DRY EYE SYNDROME

Eye doctors divide dry eye cases into one of two general types:[6]

- Fewer tears are produced. This type is called decreased tear secretion, or aqueous-deficient dry eye syndrome

- Evaporation of tears increases from the surface of the eye. This is called hyper-evaporative dry eye syndrome

ANATOMY OF DRY EYE

THREE LAYERS

The moisture-laden surface of the eye contains three interrelated layers known as the **tear film**. Stable continuity of that surface and the production of tears rely on the function of these three layers, which need to be produced in proper balanced amounts by the body to avoid dry eye syndrome.

1. The innermost layer of the surface of the eye is a **mucous layer** that forms the bulk of the tears and contains electrolytes, a variety of proteins, and water. It also has some anti-microbial properties.

2. On top, on the outside of the mucous layer, is a mildly alkaline **aqueous layer** (watery) comprising up to 90% of the thickness of the tear film.

3. Outside the watery layer is an oily **lipid layer** that slows evaporation of the tear film. This thin layer is made up of meibum, produced by the meibomian gland.

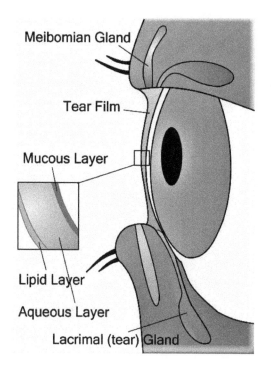

Meibomian Gland

Tear Film

Mucous Layer

Lipid Layer

Aqueous Layer

Lacrimal (tear) Gland

MUCOUS MEMBRANE

The mucous layer is the innermost layer of the tear film, closest to the surface of the cornea. "Goblet cells," floating in the conjunctiva, are gland-like cells that produce mucin. Mucin interacts with the watery layer of the tear film to form the thin mucous layer of the tear film that coats the cornea and allows for even distribution of the tear film. Goblet cells can be stimulated to elicit greater production of mucin when the eye is irritated by environmental pollutants. Irritants such as some solvents can destroy goblet cells.

Eye surgery, which holds the eyelids open, can damage the conjunctiva and destroy goblet cells. This may be why many patients experience severe dry eyes after eye surgery.

THE TEAR GLANDS

The aqueous (watery) layer makes up to 90% of the thickness of the tear film. It is created by lacrimal glands, one for each eye, which lie along the orbit (bone) of the eyes above the lateral (outside) part of the eye. The slightly alkaline (pH-7.4) liquid produced by the lacrimal glands flows through canals into the lacrimal sac that is located on the inside of each eye beside the bridge of the nose. The action of blinking pumps tears onto and across the surface of the eye. In addition, tears flow from this sac into the nose. This is the reason you get a runny nose when there is too much fluid to stay on the surface of the eyes.

Nerves connect to the lacrimal glands, providing sensory stimulation (as when you cut an onion) to stimulate tears. Blood vessels also connect to the lacrimal glands, distributing nutrients and oxygen to the gland. These glands are also tied to the lymph system and as such, help drain toxins and impurities from the surface of the eye.

Meibomian Glands

A very thin oily (lipid) layer covers the outside of the tear film and helps slow evaporation of moisture. The meibomian glands secrete meibum. They are located on the upper and lower eyelids between the eye lashes. Meibum is also produced by the Zeis and Moll glands. Meibum is fluid at body temperature. It slows tear film evaporation and lowers tear-film surface tension so that the tear film remains contoured to the surface of the eye and tears don't spill down to the cheeks. When the eyelids are closed, it is meibum that makes the eye within airtight.

BLINK FUNCTION

The normal blinking process acts as a pump on the lacrimal sac to move more fluid to the eye and distribute it across the surface of the eye. Blinking brings material from the watery and oily layers and helps to remove debris. It is an essential part of eye comfort because the tear film naturally begins to degrade after about 10 seconds and needs renewal. Therefore, we normally blink automatically about 10-12 blinks a minute. When you are focused intently on something, your blink rate slows, as when working on the computer, which can result in dry eye syndrome.

After about 10 unblinking seconds, tear film becomes unstable, leading to tired, dry eyes. This is also partially true when the blink is incomplete and does not fully cover the cornea. The cornea tells the brain to send messages to the body to produce more or fewer tears and when to blink.

SYMPTOMS

Symptoms of dry eye syndrome may include:

- Dryness and irritation
- Grittiness and a feeling that something is in your eye
- Burning and itching
- The seeming contradiction of excessive watering or tearing

RISK FACTORS AND CAUSES

Meibomian dysfunction. Most dry eye symptoms have to do with meibomian gland dysfunction (MGD).[7] This occurs when natural oil produced by the lacrimal gland is either (a) blocked by the ducts along the upper and lower lids (25–30 in each lid), or (b) blocked along the openings at the lid margin. These oils produce the top layer of the tear film called the oil layer. When these are not secreted properly, tears evaporate more quickly causing dry eyes.

Tear film changes. Any condition that reduces the production, alters the composition, or impedes the distribution of the tear film may result in dry eyes. A problem with the eyelid can prevent the tears from distributing over the eyes properly.

Computer use. Mucin 5AC is a key component of the mucous layer and is essential in protecting the ocular surface by removing debris.[8] Workers spending the most time on the computer have the lowest concentrations of mucin 5AC, which contributes to dry eye syndrome.[9]

Autoantibodies. Neutrophils are a type of immune cell which produce web-like structures across the surface of the cornea. These are known as neutrophil extracellular traps (NETs), and their function is to trap bacteria and kill them. However sometimes NETs trigger autoantibody production, antibodies that impact body's proteins. They may play a role in causing inflammation.[10]

Inflammation. Dry eye syndrome is considered to be an inflammatory condition. The "vicious cycle of chronic inflammation" is a major contributor to dry eye syndrome.[11] In Sjogren's syndrome the entire lacrimal gland that is responsible for 90% of tear production may be destroyed by inflammatory lymphocytes. Drops that may decrease inflammation are often used along with specific supplements.

Hormonal levels. Dry eyes can be a health problem, and mainly for women seems to be related to fluctuations in hormone levels, particularly estrogen and androgens. Pregnant women, women who use birth control pills, and peri-menopausal, menopausal, and also post-menopausal women frequently report dry eyes.

Aging. Dry eyes also can be an isolated problem. As we age, our eyes produce about 40% less lubrication; seniors naturally have drier eyes. Free radicals are partly to blame; they take their toll over time, damaging body tissues and increasing the prevalence of dry eye symptoms.

Contact lenses. Long-term contact lens use, especially soft lens, also can contribute to dry eyes,[12] because over time, contact lenses can reduce corneal sensitivity. The sensitivity of the cornea and the entire ocular surface determines how many tears the lacrimal gland will secrete. The less sensitive the cornea, the fewer tears or more in some cases.

Environmental issues. Tobacco smoke, environmental allergens, air conditioning, and wind might also cause dry eyes. A 5-year study showed that cigarette smokers were more likely to have dry eyes by a factor of 1.44 compared to sex and age-matched nonsmokers.[13]

Medications. Many medications trigger dry eyes, most commonly antihistamines, codeine, decongestants, diuretics, morphine, oral contraceptives, and even eyedrops such as Visine and Murine used for "getting the red out."

Migraines. Researchers have long suspected that there may be a connection between dry eyes and migraine headaches. One study investigates that tie by investigating the relationship between tear capacity and migraine symptoms in patients.[14]

Other health conditions. Like most eye conditions, dry eye syndrome often is related to health conditions in the rest of the body. It is commonly associated with dryness of other mucous membranes and brittle nails.

Dry eye syndrome also can be a sign of digestive imbalances or of more serious autoimmune diseases such as rheumatoid arthritis, Sjogren's syndrome, or lupus erythematosus. Such diseases trigger an immune response generating lymphocytes (white blood cells) that slowly destroy the cells that are responsible for tear production and secretion. As a result, tear volume decreases, cells in the conjunctiva decrease, and corneal cells can be lost. This can create dry spots.

In post-menopausal women, dry eyes also can be a sign of Sjogren's syndrome, commonly misdiagnosed. In Sjogren's syndrome, dry eyes are normally accompanied by dryness in other parts of the body: dry mouth, dry joints (arthritis), sore throat, dry skin, dry cracked lips, dry scalp (dandruff), and brittle nails. This is an autoimmune process in which antibodies attack fluid secreting cells and produce this pattern of symptoms. Fatigue and dental cavities often are present.

CONVENTIONAL APPROACH

First, a careful review is done on the patient history. Then diagnostic testing measures how salty the tear content is (osmolarity). Schirmer testing measures this tear volume. InflammaDry is a rapid in-office test that detects MMP-9, an inflammatory marker that is consistently elevated in the tears of patients with the dry eye disease. Standard medical treatment for dry eyes includes the following options: artificial tear preparations in the form of eyedrops or a procedure called punctal occlusion after which you retain more tears in your eyes by reducing tear drainage.

Treatment often includes Blephex, an instrument used to scrub the bacterial biofilm across the eyelid where approximately 50 gland openings are, probing glands as necessary, and MiBoflo treatment. MiBoflo is a 108 degree, heated, double pad with ultrasound gel to heat the lids and melt lipids, so that they flow thru the openings. With this system, eyedrops can be customized for each patient.

Sometimes the eye doctor will prescribe eyedrops such as Restasis or Xiidra for helping, over time, to produce more tears. These eyedrops can be helpful, but do have potential side effects, so these should be discussed with your eye doctor. For the more severe dry eye problems, many doctors use an amniotic membrane on the eye for healing purposes, such as Prokera.

ARTIFICIAL TEARS

Although many people find temporary relief by using artificial tear preparations, these merely temporarily relieve the symptoms. Worse, the preservatives in many of these products can aggravate the condition and can even kill corneal cells. Eyedrops called vasoconstrictors that promise to "get the red out" reduce circulation in the eye, decrease production of the tear film, and eventually make your eyes even drier. Once the effects of the vasoconstrictors wear off, the blood vessels that were constricted redilate, causing a "rebound red eye" that can trap you in a cycle of constantly having to use the drops.

PUNCTAL OCCLUSION

Many people tire of using eyedrops and turn to punctal occlusion that might provide longer-term relief. This is a procedure based on the theory that if the tear outflow is limited by occluding (blocking) the area from which the tears flow, the amount of tearing will increase. This, in turn, increases the overall length of time that tears are in contact with the cornea and may be more comfortable to dry-eye sufferers.

Punctal occlusion closes the drain that draws away excess fluids from the eyes. Here is how it works: there are tear drainage canals on the margins of the upper and lower eyelids near the nose. Tiny pumps inside the drainage opening suck away fluid from the surface of the eyes.

In punctal occlusion, the doctor closes the drain with silicone plugs, which keep most of the fluids from being pumped away. In one mega study analysis the conclusion was that plug placement resulted in ≥50% improvement of the symptoms, improvement in ocular-surface health, reduction in artificial tear use, and this improved contact lens comfort in patients with dry eye. Serious complications from plugs were infrequent.[15]

HOME TREATMENT

Also utilized is a home treatment including heat goggles and occasionally moisture goggles. Information can be collected using digital photography and video, to show the patient the difference prior to, and after, treatment.

Cyclosporine and Lifitegrast are prescription medications approved by the United States Food and Drug Administration for treating dry eyes. Corticosteroid eyedrops may be prescribed short-term to reduce eye inflammation.[16] New formulations of eye lubricant drops contain substances such as hyaluronic acid (absorbs up to 10 times its weight in water), vitamin A, E, and omega-3 oils.

Natural Eye Care: Dry Eye Syndrome

COMPLEMENTARY APPROACH

Only use eyedrops without preservatives. These have been shown to enhance corneal healing and improve dry eye problems. Several recommended brands are Thera Tears, Oasis Plus, Natural Ophthalmics' Tear Stimulation Forte eyedrops, and/or Similisan #1, 2, or 3. Thera Tears has been shown to aid in the healing of dry eyes after eight weeks of treatment. In several studies, users have reported 90% improvement. Similisan and Natural Ophthalmics have homeopathic formulations that help stimulate the eyes to produce tears naturally. We recommend eyedrops that not only help relieve dry eyes but have the potential to contribute to eye healing.

As dry eye syndrome is often related to other issues, using only eyedrops can help relieve symptoms, but it can also be extremely important to take supplements. Supplements can help internally moisten the body related to dry eyes, as well as reduce inflammation that may be related to dry eye symptoms. Some supplements help with natural tear production as well.

NUTRIENTS

★★★★ ESSENTIAL

★★★★Omega-3 fatty acids. 3,000 IU–4,500 IU per day. In an evaluation of diet and dry-eye incidence in nearly 40,000 people, researchers noted that high intakes of omega-3s taken in foods (like fish) contribute as much as 66% reduction in dry eye syndrome. These women ate 5–6 servings of tuna weekly.[17] Other subjects receiving omega-3 supplementation showed significantly reduced osmolarity. Additionally, tear break up time (TBUT) was reduced, which is a measure of how fast the tear film protecting the surface of the cornea begins to break up. Lowered levels of inflammation were observed. Of particular interest was that many of the signs and symptoms of chronic dry eye improved relatively quickly, as early as six weeks.[18]

Note 1. We do not recommend 5-6 servings of tuna weekly as these fish may contain high levels of mercury and there are other ways such as taking supplements from low level fish including sardines and mackerel.

Note 2. Because of mixed results in research, more analysis needs to be done. Eating whole fish, and paying attention to the omega-3 and omega-6 ratio may be important. One double-blind study involving about 350 people found that taking only omega-3 fatty acids did not, by itself, improve dry eye.[19]

★★★★Homeopathic eyedrops for dry eyes. In particular, homeopathic eyedrops containing the herb Cineraria Maritima has been used for decades to help manage and even potentially improve cataracts, particularly in the early stages.

★★★★Preservative free eyedrops help keep the eyes lubricated.

★★★★Castor oil eyedrops (used before bedtime) help to keep the eyes lubricated and have natural anti-inflammatory and healing properties. They are good for dry eyes symptoms particularly for those that are more severe during the night and early morning.

★★★★Dry eye formulas containing mucopolysaccharides (mucin complex) are sugar complexes that help with natural tear production. Mucin is the primary component of the mucous or innermost layer of the tear film.

★★★ IMPORTANT

★★★Evening primrose or black current oil taking 500mg per day. Black currant oil increases prostaglandin PGE1. PGE1 is a fatty compound with hormone-like effects that stimulates aqueous tear secretion and reduces the production of another prostaglandin, PGE2, which causes inflammation that contributes to dry eyes.[20]

★★★Vitamin D (vitamin D3 recommended). 2,000 to 5,000 IU per day. Not only is dry eye syndrome associated with low levels of vitamin D, but the evaporative type of dry eye syndrome is linked to changes in cornea structure (may be linked to vitamin D deficiency).[21] [22] [23]

★★ HELPFUL

★★Vitamin A (palmitate). 2,000 IU–5,000 IU per day. Vitamin A is an essential nutrient for the health of the epithelial cells of the eye's cornea and conjunctiva, and it is required for the manufacture of mucin, the primary component of the mucous (innermost) layer of the tear film.[24]

Note. Vitamin A is contra-indicated for those suffering from Stargardt disease. Pregnant women should not supplement with vitamin A.

★★Green tea extract. Patients with malfunctioning meibomian glands improved significantly compared to a control group when supplementing with this extract.[25]

★★Kidney yin tonic. The acupuncture Kidney meridian begins on the bottom of the foot and runs all the way up to the top of the chest. It helps with water metabolism throughout the body, supports overall energy, and helps with overall dryness (dry eyes, dry skin, dry scalp, etc.) Classic kidney tonics such as Ming Mu Di Huang Wan and Rehmannia-6 for example, are particularly recommended for women entering or currently going through menopause.

★★Liver tonic. In Chinese medicine the Liver "opens to the eyes" and supports overall eye health. It also helps with natural tear production. The Liver meridian begins at acupoint LV1 on the side of the big toe. From there, is ascends up the leg until it reaches the groin area, then bends sideways as it travels up the side of the torso and ends at LV14 on under the nipple on the chest, though internally passed through the eyes. A good classic Liver tonic patent formula that is available is Xiao Yao San (Rambling Powder).

Note: Visit a licensed acupuncturist to get specific formula recommendations and acupuncture treatments.

DIET

Japanese researchers investigated the impact of lifestyle changes on dry eye disease in office-based workers in a randomized, controlled trial over the course of two months. The interventions included in the trial included exercise, positive thinking, and healthy nutrition. Subjects were to eat foods with a low glycemic index, and decreased carbohydrates that included fish and vegetables at every meal. The company cafeteria now began to provide low glycemic index foods. At the beginning of the study period there were no differences in dry eye diagnosis between subjects and controls. But after two months the intervention group had fewer diagnosis of dry eye and indicators of dry eye improved. The intervention group also had lower rates of tired or sore eyes or "ocular fatigue."[26]

Limit or avoid sugar and artificial sweeteners. It is thought that excess sugar in one's diet results in too much glucose making its way to the eyes, making it difficult for the eyes to utilize all the glucose. This may result in more conditions of dry eye symptoms and can cause diabetes. 54.3% of diabetics suffer from dry eye syndrome.[27] Know what you are putting into your body.

Reduce (or try to eliminate) carbohydrate consumption,[28] particularly all refined carbohydrates, such as white flour, pasta, rice and white sugar. Keep all sugar consumption to a minimum (corn syrup being the worst).

Avoid toxic fats in commercial red meats, dairy products, fried foods, and hydrogenated oils (included in margarine and shortening). These fats interfere with the proper metabolism of essential fatty acids in the body and, indirectly, cause dry eye syndrome.

Gut issues may contribute to dry eye. Try taking a high-quality probiotic to replenish the healthy flora in your gut, particularly if you have been on long-term antibiotics. Once your symptoms are under control, try switching from probiotics in pill form to real food ferments such as sauerkraut, pickles, miso, kefir, kombucha, kimchi, etc. Not only do they provide a greater variety of beneficial bacteria than can be found in a pill, but they contain many vitamins and minerals.

If inflammation is a contributing factor in your dry eye, then it is imperative to look at the possibility that your gut (leaky gut) may be the source of the inflammation, as well as imbalances in gut flora. In many cases dry eye syndrome may be linked to conditions of chronic inflammation.[29]

Stay hydrated Studies [30]have shown that people with dry eyes have higher plasma osmolality (Posm), which is a measure of the body's electrolyte-water balance, compared to patients without dry eye.

When your Posm is higher, it can indicate that you may be dehydrated and that whole-body hydration is critical to improving dry eye syndrome. You need to stay hydrated throughout the day by maintaining the proper balance between electrolytes and water. Just drinking a sports drink with sodium and potassium will not give you the proper balance. You need to add to water a full complement of ionic trace minerals to maintain your body's homeostasis. (see Resource Directory for suggestion). Getting the right balance of electrolytes and water into your body's fluid systems such as the bloodstream, lymphatic system, and interstitial water may help to prevent dry eyes and maintain proper hydration.

Juicing is an excellent way to deliver nutrients to your body. By juicing your body receives more nutrients from larger quantities of food than you would eat during one sitting. The juicing discards the pulp which has little nutritional value and taxes the digestive process more than juices alone. The fiber the pulp contains can be gotten in foods with more nutrients such as by eating flaxseed, beans, peas, lentils, oats, etc. Our recommended juicing recipe includes:

- (preferably all organic) Parsley, beets, carrots, cucumber, tomatoes, persimmons, lemon, green-leafy vegetables. Choose at least 4-6 items to combine. Do not use too many carrots. You may also add your favorite fruits and vegetables.

29

DIGESTION

As we age past 40 years, our ability to produce the necessary digestive enzymes to break down the foods we eat diminishes; our body may not receive all the nutrients it needs for good vision.

Recommended. Supplementing with a good digestive enzyme such as a formula containing amylase, protease, lipase, and cellulose, about 10 to 15 minutes before each meal, supports healthy digestion. Another option is to take with meals one tablespoon of apple cider vinegar, or the juice of half a lemon diluted in a cup of water. An alternative is to use Swiss bitter herbs taken after meals.

For those with high cholesterol or circulatory problems, there are specific enzymes that should be taken on an empty stomach. These enzymes help break down debris and waste materials in tissue and blood, which can contribute to chronic inflammation and clogged blood vessels.

Recommended. Talk with your holistic health provider about including enzymes with meals such as serrapeptase and/or nattokinase.

Protein Digestion

Noting that proteins are digested in a "fast" or "slow" manner, researchers have reported that whey protein digests quickly and casein (milk) protein digests slowly. Whey protein stimulates amino acid production as well as protein synthesis without changing protein breakdown. Casein protein, on the other hand, was found to have a lesser effect of producing amino acids and other proteins, and it breaks down more slowly. For young men, the "slow" protein was more effective; for older men, the "fast" protein source, whey, was more effective in limiting protein loss.[31] Adding fats and carbohydrates to these whey or casein protein sources lessened the differences.

Most commercial whey protein is a mixture of whey and casein, which is a common immunogen. Native whey protein (by counter-flow technique) is the cleanest, most easily digested and assimilated whey protein. Whey protein has high amounts of the amino acid cysteine, which is important to help our bodies make glutathione, the most important antioxidant.

Recommended. Talk with your health provider about whether you should pay attention to these differences (an issue will be whether you are lactose-sensitive).

BIOAVAILABILITY AND COOKING METHODS

Another issue to consider is how the cooking method impacts nutrients. For example, lutein and zeaxanthin are important nutrients to maintain healthy vision. These nutrients can be obtained through supplements, but also through foods. For example, the lutein and zeaxanthin contained in scrambled eggs are less bioavailable than in boiled eggs.[32]

Lightly steamed vegetables are an effective way to help preserve the nutrients while making them easier to digest. Adding a little fat such as olive oil to the steamed vegetables will increase the absorption of fat-soluble vitamins, such as lutein, zeaxanthin, CoQ10, and vitamins A, E, D, K.

Recommended. If you get your vision nutrients only through foods and not through supplements, consult your nutritionist (and do some research) regarding the impact of various cooking methods on the specific nutrients you are targeting.

LIFESTYLE

Exercise such as a brisk daily walk is important for all eye conditions and overall health. It is well known that exercise is a critical tool in reducing age-related eye disease.[33] Several Japanese studies conclude that an increase in the level of physical activity can be an effective intervention for the prevention of and/or treatment of dry eye disease, as well as helping alleviate other disorders including pain in the neck, shoulders, and/or low back, and chronic depression.[34]

The 2018 Japanese study intervention protocol included four minutes of squats, twenty minutes walking, ten minutes stepping exercise, biking for sixteen minutes, lightly jog for ten minutes, or running for 7-8 minutes.[35]

Recommended. At a minimum, take a brisk 15-20 minute walk per day. Jogging and running are not essential but are helpful if you enjoy them. The point is to get outside every day and move around. If you are working at a desk job, full or part time, then be sure to get up and move around for a few minutes every hour or two.

Mind/body. The rapid pace of life often interferes with people taking time to care for themselves properly, and on all levels—mental, emotional, spiritual, and physical. However, proper care maximizes the mind/body connection and its inherent healing potential, which is essential for restoring and maintaining health.

Avoid blue light. Reduce exposure to artificial blue light from computer screens and cell phones. When we spend hours looking at screens we seem to forget to blink. This can exacerbate the dry eye syndrome and lead to other eye problems down the road. Even low levels of blue-light exposure (400-470nm) may induce photoreceptor and also retinal-pigment-epithelial cell damage.[36] Light-induced damage also increases with age, due to a decrease in protective enzymes such as superoxide dismutase (SOD). Artificial blue-light exposure appears to be more damaging at night than during the day.[37] There are blue-light-blocking glasses (ex: Blutech lenses or complete protection BP1550 tints) that can be worn while on the computer, as well as blue-light-blocking programs that can be downloaded to your computer and phone.

Touch the earth. Ground yourself as much as possible by allowing any part of your body (bare skin) to directly touch the ground (by walking barefooted or by gardening without gloves). This allows you access to the earth's abundant negative ions that have shown to protect us from free-radical-induced inflammation and also cellular damage. Grounding connects you to the earth's magnetic field and can protect your body from man-made EMF, UV light, and cosmic radiation.[38]

Breathing. Taking deep breaths is essential to getting oxygen into the eyes. One method is to sit or stand, and take long, slow, full breaths. Keep your stomach relaxed.

When you reach full intake, then slowly breathe out until you reach the bottom of your breath, then start again. Repeat this for a minute or two. Keep the breathing in an even flow without stopping at the top or bottom of each breath. If you work at a desk, at a computer, or if you have poor, slouched posture, the ability to obtain deep, full, cleansing breaths is more difficult, which not only affects eye health but also directly affects energy, vitality, and general health.

A good eye yoga exercise that relaxes the eye and uses breathing techniques is called Palming.

1.   Sit on a chair and keep your elbows on a table in front you.
2.   With your hands crossed overlapping each other, cover your eyes without the palms touching your eyelids.
3.   Breathe in through the diaphragm to a count of ten, keeping your stomach muscles relaxed. Hold the breath 3-5 seconds and then slowly breathe out to a count of ten. Feel the tension release. Relax.

Recommended. Consider seeing a Buteyko breath instructor to learn how to breathe properly.

OTHER MODALITIES

★CHINESE MEDICINE

Life according to Chinese philosophy is all about balance: the perfect balance of yin and yang. These concepts are thousands of years old. Chinese Medicine practitioners believed that everything in life is subject to this law of nature, which you will see exhibited in nature, often in the form of opposite forces.

Yin energy, for example, is cooling energy; it relates to sunset and nighttime, to rest and repair, and to building blood and fluids. It has "descending" energy (yin energy flows inward and downward), dominates the left side of the body, and embodies qualities of the Mother. As far as foods go, yin is the realm of salty, bitter, and sour.

Yang, on the other hand, is warming energy. It relates to morning energy, the sunrise, and also daytime activity. Yang has "ascending" energy (energy that rises outward and upward), dominates the right side of the body, and embodies qualities of the Father. In terms of foods, yang is associated with both sweet and pungent foods.

The Chinese recognized this long ago. In fact, all of Traditional Chinese Medicine (TCM) naturally works to balance yin and yang. Whether the purpose is to maintain proper body temperature, correct acid and alkaline levels in the tissue and blood, or overall harmony in the body, yin and yang are always at work. When either yin or yang becomes imbalanced, discomfort occurs. If steps are not then taken to address the underlying cause of the imbalance, pain and disease will occur. The type of disease that occurs and where it occurs in the body depends on any number of factors, in addition to the underlying condition or imbalance, such as genetics and lifestyle choices.

Although there are a number of conditions and circumstances that can result in dry eyes, acupuncture and Chinese herbal formulas often help manage the dry eye problem and reduce symptoms. What we eat affects how we feel, supports heath and balance in the body, and reduces the risk of disease onset. In Chinese medicine, balanced meridians are key; western medicine refers to it as homeostasis. Basically, when we are in balance, we can avoid disease. Being chronically out of balance eventually results in pain and disease.

Meridian balances and imbalances in TCM are related to patterns (for example, Liver Yang Rising, Yin Deficiency, Spleen Dampness, etc.). The patterns may be described as follows:

- Too much or too little yin or yang
- Too much or too little functioning of the TCM meridian systems
- Too warm or too cold

- Too moist or too dry
- Not enough qi, the flow of energy
- Movement upward or downward

The Liver "opens to the eyes" and is the primary meridian for supporting overall flow of energy and circulation through the eyes. It also helps your body with natural tear production.

The Kidney meridian nourishes the blood to the eyes and helps with internal water metabolism often related to dry eye syndrome. Other meridians may be out of balance as well that can affect eye health, so an evaluation by an acupuncturist can best determine where the out-of-balances are and offer the optimal treatment strategy. Acupuncture treatments are typically done by inserting needles below the knees and elbows, then in specific points along the orbit of the eye and under the eye (not in the eye). An evaluation by an acupuncturist is the best way to determine where the imbalances are.

All of the TCM meridian systems (organs) have patterns that pertain to ocular functioning. Some types of imbalances stand on their own; in other words, they are not "types" of yin or yang. Others are too much or too little yin or yang.

DEFICIENT LIVER AND KIDNEY YIN

Major ocular symptoms include cataracts, AMD, Stargardt's, open angle glaucoma, retinitis pigmentosa, Usher syndrome, dry eye, optic neuritis, and retinal bleeding. Retinal bleeding may be considered more of a spleen deficiency, heat, or stasis.

BLOOD DEFICIENCY

Major ocular symptoms include Stargardt's disease, floaters, dry eye, retinal vein or artery occlusion, and night blindness. Foods that help build blood include the following:

- **Vegetables.** Alfalfa sprouts, artichoke, avocado, beetroot, cabbage, celery, dandelion leaf, chlorophyll-rich foods, kelp, dark leafy-green vegetables, garlic, fresh ginger, leeks, shiitake mushroom, button mushroom, onions, spinach, watercress, wheatgrass, winter squash and pumpkin, parsnips, black sesame, and spirulina
- **Meats.** Beef, liver (both pork and sheep), bone stock/soup, chicken, oysters, and eggs
- **Grains.** Molasses, barley, corn, bran, rice, oats, sweet rice, and wheat
- **Fruit.** Apple, apricot, avocado, date, fig, grape, and goji berries

DEFICIENT YANG (Heat)

Major ocular symptoms include diabetic retinopathy, retinitis pigmentosa, Ushers syndrome, choroidal dystrophy, and optic nerve atrophy. Foods that help tonify yang include the following:

- **Fruit**. Cherries, persimmon, coconut, lemons, raspberries, blackberry, mulberry
- **Vegetables**. Cauliflower, mustard greens, beets, string beans, onion, cabbage, kale, garlic, fresh ginger, chestnuts, daily soups with onions, garlic, ginger, and leeks
- **Meats**. Chicken and turkey
- **Dairy**. Yogurt and butter
- **Grains**. Barley, wheat, rice, quinoa, amaranth, and sweet brown rice
- **Seeds and nuts**. Millet, pumpkin seeds, walnuts
- **Legumes**. Tofu, kidney beans, black beans, mung beans, and mung bean sprouts
- **Other**. Seaweeds and micro-algae (especially chlorella and spirulina)

Deficient Kidney Yang

Major ocular symptoms include diabetic retinopathy, Usher syndrome, choroidal dystrophy, optic nerve atrophy, and retinitis pigmentosa. The latter may be considered more Lung Deficiency but may also be Kidney Yang Deficiency.

EXCESSIVE YANG (HEAT)

Major ocular symptoms include wet macular degeneration, diabetic retinopathy, ocular (and regular) migraines, dry eyes, glaucoma, eyestrain, and blurry vision.

Common disorders that may show up in other areas of the body include dry skin, excessive thirst, heat intolerance, nosebleeds, high blood pressure, a rapid pulse, temple headaches, tremors, tinnitus, hearing impairment, rashes, swelling, restlessness, skin eruptions, local inflammation, inflammation in any part of the body, constipation, blood in the urine, and thick yellow or green phlegm, as with a cold or bronchitis. Foods to help reduce excess yang include the following:

- Cooling foods. Consume your consumption of cooling foods down to 10% for 30 days. Cooling foods include the following:
  - ➢ **Vegetables**: cucumber, celery, spinach, bok choy, broccoli, sweet corn, zucchini, radish, lettuce, and eggplant
  - ➢ **Fruit**: apple, cantaloupe, watermelon, pear, tomato, banana, and apples
  - ➢ **Fluids.** These should also be cooling, such as vegetable or fruit juices, broths, and herbal teas; room temperature green tea is also permitted. Ideally, beverages should be consumed at room temperature, rather than when cold. Cold foods and beverages can disrupt stomach acid, and can further weaken the body.
  - ➢ **Reduce specific foods**. Reduce red meat, chicken, coffee, alcohol, and spicy foods.

EXCESSIVE YIN (COOLING)

Major ocular symptoms include myopia, astigmatism, blurry vision, cataracts, macular degeneration, retinitis pigmentosa, diabetic retinopathy, photophobia, and/or poor night vision.

Other conditions signaling excessive yin are cold intolerance, chill sensations, body pain from cold weather conditions, copious excretions of clear body fluids such as with the onset of cold symptoms, afternoon headaches, dry stools, restlessness, poor sleep, dizziness, diabetes, tuberculosis, hypoglycemia, chronic inflammation, and infection (from viruses, parasites, bacteria, and fungi).

Excessive yin can be caused by over consumption of rich or denatured foods, which includes all fast food, processed food, and those foods high in fat and sugar. In addition, the consumption of alcohol and coffee, smoking, taking synthetic drugs (pharmaceuticals), being overly competitive, all contribute to not managing chronic stress effectively.

Blood and tissue also may be lacking in calcium, as well as other cooling minerals and even essential fatty acids (particularly omega-3 fatty acids), which help keep the arteries clean, prevent inflammation, and therefore prevent the buildup of heat. Recommended foods include the following:

- **Fruit.** Watermelon, blackberry, raspberry, grapes, banana, melons, pear, and persimmon
- **Vegetables.** Beets, string beans, spinach, leafy-green vegetables, asparagus, kuzu, and daily soups
- **Grains.** Quinoa, millet, barley, and amaranth
- **Legumes.** Black beans, mung beans, and kidney beans
- **Seafood.** Crab, anchovies, and sardines
- **Other.** Pine nuts, sprouts, microalgae, tofu, seaweed, chlorella, and spirulina
- **Avoid** spicy and overly warm foods, alcohol, coffee, and black tea

LIVER WIND

According to Traditional Chinese Medicine (TCM), many problems with the eyes are related to the health of the liver (meridian) system. Strategies to restore the liver to optimal function consequently improve eye health. Internal Liver Wind, an extreme imbalance of yin and yang, Qi and Blood can result of extreme heat within the liver. Internal liver wind may cause the eyeball to turn upwards and move involuntarily (nystagmus). Liver wind is frequently associated with severe emotional stress, vertigo, dizziness, neck stiffness and headache.

Major ocular symptoms include acute-angle closure glaucoma, open-angle glaucoma (usually not so much unless it is sudden), sudden retinal bleeding, optic neuritis, cataracts (may be more fluid deficiency and

Liver Kidney Yin deficiency), Non Arteritic Interior Ischemic Optic Neuropathy (NAION), retinal detachment, occlusions, sudden eye pain, stye, and nastagmus.

Foods that help reduce or extinguish Liver Wind include:

- Vegetables: Celery, cucumber, lettuce, watercress, basil, sage, fennel, ginger, anise, oats, black soybean, black sesame seed, mung beans and their sprouts, pine nuts, coconut, tofu, fresh cold-pressed flax oil, lemon, plum, rhubarb root, radish, and chamomile

Foods that worsen Liver Wind include:

- Eggs, crabmeat, and buckwheat
- Excessive meat in the diet can also be toxic to the liver.

DEFICIENT QI

Major ocular symptoms include retinitis pigmentosa, macular degeneration (wet and dry), Usher syndrome, and presbyopia. Foods that help build "qi" include the following:

- **Grains**. All grains including quinoa, oats, pearl barley, and brown rice
- **Meats**. Chicken and lamb
- **Legumes**. All lentils and legumes
- **Eggs**
- **Fish**

- **Vegetables**. Green beans, leeks, carrots, onion, root vegetables, potatoes, mushrooms, pumpkin and squash, soybeans, string beans, tofu, turnips, and yams
- **Fruit**. Goji berries, cherries, dates, figs, coconut and loganberry
- **Other**. Fox nut, ginseng, nutmeg, green tea, jasmine tea, and raspberry leaf tea

EXCESS DAMPNESS

Major ocular symptoms include macular degeneration (wet and dry), diabetic retinopathy, macular edema, cystoid macula edema, and central serous retinopathy.

Foods to help reduce excess dampness include;

- **Vegetables**. Organic lightly cooked vegetables, corn, celery, watercress, lettuce, turnip, pumpkin, alfalfa sprouts, button mushrooms, radish, turnip, and scallion
- **Grains**. Rye, amaranth, brown rice, barley, and oats
- **Legumes**. Adzuki beans, kidney beans, and lentils
- **Meat**. Small amount of lean organic meat, poultry, and fish
- **Fruit.** Small amount of whole fruits and lemon
- **Other**. Raw honey, all bitter herbs, sesame seeds, pumpkin seeds, sunflower seeds, wild blue-green algae, seaweed, and kelp

- **Avoid** dairy, cold raw foods, cold drinks, wheat (and refined wheat flour) for those that are gluten sensitive, peanuts and peanut butter, avocado, coffee, and alcohol. Avoid overeating.

CHINESE MEDICINE PATENT FORMULAS

- Preserve vistas pill (zhu jing wan). Tonifies and nourishes the Liver and Kidneys, enriches the yin and improves vision.

- Ming mu di huang wan (rehmannia pills to brighten the eyes). This is related to the patterns of Liver blood deficiency, Kidney yin deficiency, and/or Liver yin deficiency

- Xiao yao san (rambling powder). Classic Liver tonic that supports the flow of the Liver meridian energy.

★MENTAL BODY: MEDITATION

The goal of yoga is union with the "divine," which can also be called reality, or the Tao, the Creative Infinite, nature, "that which is," or the Universal. In yoga philosophy, the Universal is said to exist in the space between thoughts, which is non-thinking; in this infinite space, the Truth of Being is said to reside. This place of "no mind" is meditation.

Many advanced practitioners of yoga and meditation who are able to enter the "space between thoughts" report improved vision afterwards. To quote Michael Hutchison from *The Book of Floating*, "As I went out into the world [after going into the state of no mind] my senses were extremely—almost unbelievably—sharp and keen. Everything I saw seemed beautiful and miraculous, and the colors of everything were extraordinarily rich and beautiful. I saw everything clearly, as if objects had sharp edges around. Everything has become much sharper and clearer than it normally was."

The takeaway here is that external vision can be improved as you raise your level of consciousness. In other words, meditation and deepening your meditation practice (i.e. inner vision) can be a doorway to improving your eyesight (outer vision).

There are many meditation methods, but all aim to quiet the mind and bring it to focus and concentration, to the place of "no mind."

One yoga meditation technique works directly with the eyes. It is named trataka, and according to the *Hatha Yoga Pradipika*, one of the earliest texts on hatha yoga, trataka is said to eradicate all eye diseases, fatigue, and sloth, and to close the doorway creating these problems. In addition to improving concentration and memory, trataka cleanses both the eyes and the cerebral cortex, balances the nervous system, and relieves depression, anxiety, and insomnia. Another yogic text, the *Gheranda Samhita*, states that the practice cultivates clairvoyance and inner vision.

Trataka has to do with gazing or fixing the eyes on one point, either on an object or often on a candle flame. In a scientific study performed at Svyasa University, Bengaluru, India, and published in 2014, one month of trataka intervention "improved cognitive functions [short-term and working memory, selective and focused attention, concentration, visual scanning, and activation and inhibition of rapid responses and executive functions] when compared to wait-list control group."[39]

Stress is often a big factor in contributing to poorer vision and even eye disease. Meditation and relaxation techniques are increasingly recognized for their value in reducing stress.[40] [41]There are several main types of meditation, and each provide comfort and value,[42] depending on your own style of functioning, how much time you can make for your practice, and whether the practice requires a quiet place.

Focused attention (FA). Trataka is an example of a focused meditation in which you focus your attention on one single object. If you live a very relaxed life, then this technique may help sharpen your attention.[43] Trataka requires sitting cross-legged, with a straight back and a candle at the level of your eyes. This form has been found to support improved vision.[44]

Open monitoring (OM). Buddhist mindfulness techniques are good examples in which you contemplate breath or thoughts in order to detach from being controlled by them. Open monitoring techniques have been found to produce beneficial mental and physical health outcomes. In experienced practitioners measured brain patterns in the frontal lobe are found to powerfully change during this practice.[45]

Automatic self-transcending (AST). Transcendental meditation (TM) and vedic meditation are examples, in which no concentration/contemplation is used, but which yield qualitatively different end results. These are good techniques if you live a demanding, stressful life. They have been found to produce good physical outcomes, especially reducing anxiety, addiction, hypertension, sleeplessness, and migraines. As in OM techniques, frontal lobe activity changes; in addition, alpha functioning improves across the brain.[46]

★HERBAL TEA

Chrysanthemum and goji berry tea. Chrysanthemum flowers have heat-clearing properties that are so important in helping cool off red, dry eyes. Goji berries are beneficial for the kidneys, the lungs, the liver, and build yin fluids such as tears. Brew the chrysanthemum flowers like you would any loose tea and then put a small handful of goji berries into the made tea. After drinking the tea, you can eat the berries

★ESSENTIAL OILS

- **Carrot seed** essential oil has antiseptic, disinfectant, detoxifier, and antioxidant properties.

- **Frankincense** helps relieve chronic stress and anxiety, reduces pain and inflammation, and boosts immunity.

- **Clary sage** helps balance the endocrine system.

Combine ¼ cup of avocado oil with ¼ cup of calendula-infused oil. Slowly add 5 drops each of the essential oils. Then close the bottle and shake well; apply 4 drops of this mixture on your clean face. Massage in gentle circular motions. Leave overnight.

Note: Keep essences away from the mouth, eyes, and mucous membranes; if a few drops get in one of these sensitive areas it may be uncomfortable for 15–30 minutes, but not harmful. You can lessen discomfort by adding a pure oil like olive or coconut oil to neutralize the irritating effect. For the eye area, dab a few drops around the outside of the eye. Do not put the neutralizing oil in the eye.

VISUAL HYGIENE

Headaches, squinting, and eyes that burn, ache, water, or tire easily are indications that the visual system needs help. Most people are born with the potential for good eyesight. Vision, however, is learned. And the way you use and care for your visual system directly affects your success at school or work and enjoyment of play. Your visual system can undergo tremendous stress.

CHANGING VISION NEEDS

Students now read three times the number of textbooks their grandparents did. Though book reading can lead to eyestrain, textbooks are becoming anachronistic as we shift to digital texts and other digital learning software, which has its own problems in vision.[47] Children and teens are increasingly relying on digital materials at school and they are obsessing with digital games, social media, and more, which is leading to additional serious consequences in vision health. Some children start looking at electronic screens from infancy.

Although parents may be familiar with vision damage from UVA and UVB light from the sun, few are aware of the damage to the retina from blue light, which is emitted by the digital screens of electronic devices and fluorescent and LED lighting.

The most common visual problems that are reported among college-aged computer users were headache

(53.3%), burning sensation in the eyes (54.8%), and tired eyes (48%).[48] While studies on the effects of computer eyestrain are not yet prevalent, taking a look at data related to repetitive strain injuries (RSIs) can help put this problem in perspective.

Adults constantly use near vision at work and play. The shift to computers has engaged a growing number of workers in prolonged, near-vision tasks. Eye discomfort, headaches, blurred vision, lowered visual performance, and a wide array of vision-linked problems are related to this heavy, near-point vision overload, not to mention increased risk of glaucoma,[49] [50] dry eye,[51] advanced macular degeneration, damage to rods and cones[52] and the retinal pigmented layer of macula,[53] and eye cancer.[54] One study showed excess computer use could result in a 40% reduction of work productivity.[55]

In addition to the direct physical damage from blue light emitted from electronic screens, the slumped physical position that the body adopts causes indirect damage to the eyes and body. Prolonged hunching over a computer terminal increases neck-muscle tightness, which causes neuro-vascular compression, reduces available oxygen and nutrients, and impinges on nerve conduction to and from the body and the head. Additionally, this position compresses the lung cavities, preventing full, nourishing breathing.

HUNTER-SOLDIER EYES

The problem is that human beings were not designed to do constant viewing within an arm's length away. We evolved hunter-soldier eyes for survival and spotting game and enemies at a distance. Only in the last half-century have so many people been forced to deal with sustained, near-visual tasks. The result has been a constant stress on the visual system that we were not designed to endure, producing eye symptoms and related problems. Many vision and eye problems are the direct result of an adaptation (or failure to adapt) to these relatively new, near-centered visual tasks. It's no wonder that ignoring good visual hygiene, the impact of long-term visual stress, or the failure to heed symptoms of vision problems can have a significant effect on the quality and enjoyment of a person's life.

MORE THAN 20/20

The standard eye test uses the Snellen chart, which was designed around 1860 to test students' ability to read a chalkboard from the back of a schoolroom; it indicates distance visual acuity (clarity of sight).

The Snellen chart does not test the ability of a person to handle near-visual work such as reading, writing, or prolonged close-up activities — "near-point vision." Near-point visual stress, despite 20/20 distance clarity, has been shown to lead to the development of visual problems and eye conditions, including dry eyes[56] (often the result of a reduced blinking rate), increased myopia,[57] and glaucoma.[58] Blurred vision, dry eyes, burning sensation, redness of eyes, headache as well as visual fatigue symptoms such as sore eyes and increased glare sensitivity[59] are the main symptoms resulting from improper use of computer.[60] Myopia (nearsightedness) is one of these eye conditions. Between 1999 and 2004, approximately 41.6% of the population of the United States was diagnosed as nearsighted, compared to 25% measured and assessed between the years 1971–1972; that is a 16.6% increase in three decades. Myopia now appears at earlier ages., Usually the earlier it appears, the deeper the person advances into nearsightedness. Increasingly strong lenses for distance vision are required as myopia progresses. Another treatment option is to work with a vision therapist to help to maintain your prescription and possibly reduce it. Daily exercising and taking regular breaks from reading and computer use to do these eye exercises can help maintain strong, healthy vision.

The most common result of visual stress is lowered achievement as mentioned in the study above. When chronic stress is present, people usually do one of several things:

- Avoid the task by doing as little as you can to get by.
- Experience pain or other symptoms (such as aches, visual or body fatigue, and falling asleep when reading).

- Suppress the sight of one eye at the cost of reduced efficiency and understanding.
- Develop myopia or astigmatism.
- Get frustrated because of difficulty concentrating.
- Strain harder to get the work or reading done.
- Any combination of the above

TAKE BETTER CARE OF YOUR VISION

Below we list some basic guidelines for reducing visual stress.

Looking up. Both children and adults need to look up and away from near tasks to distant objects regularly. From a Chinese medicine perspective, electronic devices give off "fire" (not actual fire) energy. So, when looking at computer or cell phone screens, it would help to look far away, every 30 minutes, to something green, like trees.

Lighting. The illumination on what you are doing should be three times brighter than the rest of the room. Don't read under a single lamp in a dark room. Eliminating glare is especially important for close-up work. Lighting should not be fluorescent or LED as they have an unbalanced color spectrum, too strong in the blue range, which can contribute to impaired sleep in the short term and to retinal damage in the long run. Additionally, fluorescent lights flicker at a rate that is undetectable to the human eye and can cause eyestrain and dizziness. Incandescent lighting is the better choice. Try to avoid exposure to bright lights, computer screens, and cell phones at least 3–4 hours before sleep.

Sitting straight. Have chest up, shoulders back, and weight over the seat so both eyes are at the eye task level and at an equal distance from what is being seen.

Best distance. Reading, writing, or close-up work is best done at an eye-to-activity distance equal to the length between middle knuckle and elbow (14–16 inches for adults).

Posture. Sit upright while reading or watching television in bed. Avoid lying on your back or stomach.

Writing. Hold your pencil or pen an inch or so from the tip so you can see and guide it without tilting your head or body to the side.

Screen time. Watch TV from a distance equal to seven times the width of the screen (about eight to ten feet) and sit upright. Have indirect lamps on in the room but placed to eliminate glare on the screen. Watching television involves and develops very few visual skills and should be limited to a few hours or less daily, especially for children. Computer screens should be placed at least 2-3 feet away from your eyes to reduce the effect of the electromagnetic fields and blue light.

Participating. Perform outdoor activities that require seeing at a distance. Become aware of what and where things are on all sides. When walking, keep your head up, eyes wide open, and look toward objects but avoid staring at them.

NOURISHING YOUR EYES

Medical science doesn't really know why or how most poor eyesight develops. It wrongly believes that eyesight can only worsen; that once eyesight starts to go, nothing can be done about it, and that all we can do is stand by idly and watch it deteriorate. The good news is that we don't have to be passive victims of deteriorating eyesight. The following information from a variety of approaches can help preserve your gift of sight. Good nutrition, physical exercise, and recommended eye exercises all support your vision. Other health modalities, including acupuncture, spinal adjustments, massage, and craniosacral work, can also help your vision.

NUTRITION

When Mom and Dad told you to eat your carrots because they were good for your eyes, they were on the right track. Researchers are continually documenting that we really are what we eat. The role of nutrition and its effect on the eyes undoubtedly plays a key role.

It is believed that more than 25% of the nutrients we absorb from our food nourishes our "visual system," which includes our eyes, nerves, blood vessels, and the tissues that support our vision. The concentration of vitamin C in healthy eyes is higher than almost anywhere else in the body. A good diet, high in fruits and vegetables along with supplementation of lutein, zeaxanthin, bilberry, and vitamin A, is beneficial for keeping the eyes healthy. Additional nutrients may be required for specific eye conditions.

Inflammation

Chronic inflammation causes increased production of free radicals in the body and oxidative stress. Antioxidants reduce oxidative stress, neutralize free radicals, and many reduce inflammation.

EXERCISE

Aerobic exercise not only benefits your heart, but it is good for your eyes. Exercise is extremely important in preventing your eyes from worsening. It raises oxygen levels in the cells and increases lymph and blood circulation. Increased circulation is a necessary prerequisite for good vision.

We recommend that you gently build up to aerobic exercise for a minimum of 20 minutes per day, four days per week. You don't have to join a health club, run five miles a day, or bench press 300 pounds to have good vision. The following are some great ways of staying in shape and helping to maintain healthy eyes:

- **Walking or jogging**. Get a good, comfortable, supportive pair of walking or jogging shoes, and select a route that won't have you pounding concrete (which is bad for your joints).

- **Rebounding**. A rebounder is a mini-trampoline. Rebounding is gentle jumping on a trampoline. This exercise keeps blood flowing and improves circulation, particularly in the legs and head. Rebounding is also a great way to stimulate the lymphatic system, which removes toxins from the body.

- **Jumping rope**. This childhood activity is actually a wonderful way to stay in shape and only requires a jump rope and 5–10 minutes per day.

- **Eye exercises.** Everyone knows that you have to exercise muscles in order to keep them fit. This applies not only to heart, leg, and arm muscles, but to eye muscles as well. To improve visual fitness, you need to regularly exercise your eye muscles.

  Note: A free book on how to do these exercises is mentioned in the Resource Directory at the end of this book.

- **Earthing.** This is an inexpensive and easy way to reduce inflammation in the eyes and body. By simply walking barefoot on grass or sand, you will absorb negative electrons from the earth. Additionally, grounding can be achieved by purchasing grounding bedsheets to be used during sleep and mats to be used while on the computer or while watching TV.

ON THE HORIZON

The MiBoFlo Thermoflo is a therapeutic device providing an alternative therapy for dry eyes. This device uses a proprietary thermoelectric heat pump to help maximize liquefaction of meibum, thus improving the preservation and function of the evaporative component of the tear film. This therapy is aimed at improving function of the meibomian component of the tear film.

A small pilot study and a later randomized, double-blind, placebo-controlled trial were done. They both found that a standardized maqui berry extract increased tear production and relieved dry eye.[61] [62]

With the understanding that DNA webs (NETs) may be responsible or contribute to dry eye disease, research suggests that human globulin, pooled from thousands of adult donors, and used in eye drop form may reduce signs and symptoms.[63]

A phase I/II clinical trial of an enzyme-based treatment for severe dry shows promise. It uses a synthetic form of the DNase enzyme. Normally enzymes clear up DNA and other debris from the surface of the cornea, but in dry eye patients, DNase is deficient.[64]

These are just a few of the avenues of investigation. To see more, go to pubmed.ncbi.nlm.nih.gov and search for dry eye (along with any other keywords that interest you). -*Contributor: Ammi Ranani, OD*

RESOURCE/SUPPLEMENTS

Sample products for lens and over eye support:

- Women's Tear Stimulation Homeopathic eyedrops (or pellets that dissolve by mouth) – helps lubricate the eyes and promotes natural tear production.
- Tear Stimulation Forte Homeopathic eyedrops (or pellets that dissolve by mouth) – helps lubricate the eyes and promotes natural tear production. For overall general population
- Hylatears Eyedrops – preservative free eyedrop with glycerine and sodium hyaluronate
- Oasis PF (Preservative Free) Eyedrops - preservative free eyedrop.
- Dr. Grossman's MaxiTears Gelcaps Capsules - Helps internally moisten the body and helps with natural tear production.
- Dr. Grossman's Omega-7 Chronic Dry Eye and Anti-Inflammatory Formula - Omega-7 Fish Oil for dry eyes and inflammation symptoms.
- Eye Doctor Plus Reusable Moist Heat Compress Treatment Pack – can be heated either thru a microwave or oven.
- Castor Oil eyedrops (1 drop in each eye at bedtime) for more severe dry eye issues, particularly worse at night.

- electroBlast™ electrolyte concentrate. Add to purified water to restore full-spectrum ionic trace minerals to your drink.
- OPTASE® Dry Eye INTENSE Drops (.58 fl. oz.) - for moderate to severe dry eyes
- OPTASE® Eyelid Wipes - with tea tree oil, aloe, chamomile, hyaluronic acid and more.
- OPTASE® Dry Eye Spray (.58 fl. oz)
- Eye exercise booklet mentioned on page 61 is available at no charge on the website: www.NaturalEyeCare.com

These products can be found at www.naturaleyecare.com

Email: info@naturaleyecare.com
Phone: 845-475-4158

ENDNOTES

[1] Sharma, A., Hindman, H.B. (2014). Aging: a predisposition to dry eyes. *J Ophthalmol,* 2014:781683.

[2] Azcarate, P.M., Venincasa, V.D., Feuer, W., Stanczyk, F., Shally, A.V., Galor, A. (2014). Androgen deficiency and dry eye syndrome in the aging male. *Invest Ophthalmol Vis Sci,* Jul 3;55(8):5046-53.

[3] Ding, J., Sullivan, D.A., (2012). Aging and dry eye disease. *Exp Gerontol,* Jul;47(7):483-90.

[4] O'Brien, P.D., Collum, L.M. (2004). Dry eye: diagnosis and current treatment strategies. *Curr Allergy Asthma Rep,* 4:314–319.

[5] Schaumberg, D.A., Sullivan, D.A., Buring, J.E., Dana, M.R. (2003). Prevalence of dry eye syndrome among US women. *Am J Ophthalmol,* Aug; 136(2):318-26.

[6] Messmer, E.M. (2015). The Pathophysiology, Diagnosis, and Treatment of Dry Eye Disease. *Dtsch Arztebl Int.* Jan 30;112(5):71-81.

[7] Nowinska, A., Wylegala, E., Tarnawska, D., Janiszewska, D., Dobrowolskia, D. (2012). Meibomian gland dysfunction—review. *Klin Oczna,* 114(2):147-52.

[8] Gipson, I.K., Hori, Y., Argueso, P. (2004). Character of ocular surface mucins and their alteration in dry eye disease. *Ocul Surf,* 2(2):131-148.

[9] Uchino, Y., Uchino, M., Yokoi, N. (2014). Alteration of Tear Mucin 5AC in Office Workers Using Visual Display Terminals: The Osaka Study. *JAMA Ophthalmol,* 132(8):985-992.

[10] An, S., Raju, I., Surenkhuu, B., Kwon, J.E., Gulati, S., et al. (2019). Neutrophil Extracellular Traps (NETs) Contribute to Pathological Changes of Ocular Graft-Vs-Host Disease (oGVHD) Dry Eye: Implications for Novel Biomarkers and Therapeutic Strategies. *Ocul Surf.* Jul;17(3):589-614.

[11] Yamaguchi, T. (2018). Inflammatory Response in Dry Eye. *Invest Ophthalmol Vis Sci,* 2018 Nov 1;59(14):DES192-DES199.

[12] Kastelan, S., Lukenda, A., Salpek-Rabatic, J., Pavan, J., Gotovac, M. (2013). Dry eye symptoms and signs in long-term contact lens wearers. *Coll Antropol,* Apr;37 Suppl 1:199-203

[13] Moss, S.E., Klein, R., Klein, B.E. (2000). Prevalence of and risk factors for dry eye syndrome. *Arch Ophthalmol,* Sep; 118(9):1264-8.

[14] Koktekir, B.E., Celik, G., Karalezli, A., Kal, A. (2012). Dry eyes and migraines: Is there really a correlation? *Cornea,* Dec;31(12):1414-6.

[15] Marcet, M.M., Shtein, R.M., Bradley, E.A., Deng, S.X., Meyer, D.R., et al. (2015). Safety and efficacy of

lacrimal drainage system plugs for dry eye syndrome. *Ophthalmology*, Aug;122(8):1681-7.

[16] National Eye Institute, Facts about dry eye. Retrieved Dec 17 2017 from nei.nih.gov/health/dryeye/dryeye.

[17] Epitropoulous, A.T., Donnenfeld, E.D., Shah, Z.A., Holland, E.J., Gross, M., et al. (2016). Effect of Oral Re-esterified Omega-3 Nutritional Supplementation on Dry Eyes. *Cornea*, Sep;35(9):1185-91.

[18] Miljanovic, B., Trivedi, K.A., Dana, M.R., Gilbard, J.P., Buring, J.E., et al. (2005). Relation between dietary n-3 and n-6 fatty acids and clinically diagnosed dry eye syndrome in women. *Am J Clin Nutr*, Oct;82(4):887-93.

[19] Dry Eye Assessment and Management Study Research Group. (2018). n−3 Fatty Acid Supplementation for the Treatment of Dry Eye Disease. *N Engl J Med,* Apr 13.

[20] Baudouin, C. (1986). Dry eye: An unexpected inflammatory disease. Arch Soc *Esp Oftalmol*, 76: 205-206.

[21] Shetty, R. Sethu, S., Deshmukh, R., Despande, K., Ghosh, A., et al. (2016). Corneal dendritic cell density is associated with sub-basal nerve plexus features, ocular surface disease index, and serum vitamin D in evaporative dry eye disease. *BioMed Res Int*, 2016:4369750.

[22] Denurcum, G., Karaman, E.S., Ozsutcu, M., Eliacik, M., Olmuscelik, O., et al. (2016). Dry eye assessment in patients with vitamin D deficiency. *Eye Contact Lens*, Sep 22.

[23] Nejabat, M., Reza, S.A., Zadmehr, M., Yasemi, M., Sobhani, Z. (2017). Efficacy of green tea extract for treatment of dry eye and meibomian gland dysfunction; A double-blind randomized controlled clinical trial study. *J Clin Diagn Res*, Feb;11(2):NC05-NC08.

[24] Tei, M., Spurr-Michaud, S.J., Tisdale, A.S., Gipson, I.K. (2000). Vitamin A deficiency alters the expression of mucin genes by the rat ocular surface epithelium. *Invest Ophthalmol Vis Sci*, Jan;41(1):82-8.

[25] Ibid. Nejabat. (2017).

[26] Kawashima, M., Sano, K., Takechi, S., Tsubota, K. (2018). Impact of lifestyle intervention on dry eye disease in office workers: a randomized controlled trial. *J Occup Health.* Jul 20;60(4):281-288.

[27] Masoud, R.M., Rashidi, M., Afkhami-Ardekani, M., Shoja, M.R. (2008). Prevalence of dry eye syndrome and diabetic retinopathy in type 2 diabetic patients. *BMC Ophthalmol*, Jun 2;8:10.

[28] Ibid. Kawashima. (2018).

[29] Ibid. Baudouin. (1986).

[30] Neil P. Walsh; Matthew B. Fortes; Philippa Raymond-arker; Claire Bishop; Julian Owen; Emma Tye; Marieh Esmaeelpour; Christine Purslow; Salah Elghenzai Is Whole-Body Hydration an Important Consideration in Dry Eye? Cornea | September 2012

[31] Dangin, M., Boirie, Y., Guillet, C., Beaufrere, B. (2002). Influence of the protein digestion rate on protein turnover in young and elderly subjects. *J Nutr,* Oct;132(10):3228S-33S.

[32] Nimalaratne, C., Savard, P., Gauthier, S.F., Schieber, A., Wu, J. (2015). Bioaccessibility and digestive stability of carotenoids in cooked eggs studied using a dynamic in vitro gastrointestinal model. *J Agric Food Chem,* Mar 25;63(11):2956-62.

[33] Pardue, M.T., Chrenek, M.A., Schmidt, R.H., Nickerson, J.M., Boatright, J.H. (2015). Potential Role of Exercise in Retinal Health. *Prog Mol Biol Transl Sci,* 134:491-502.

[34] Kawashima, M., Uchino, M., Yokoi, N., Uchino, Y., Dogru, M., et al. (2014). The Association between dry eye disease and physical activity as well as sedentary behavior: Results from the Osaka study. *J Ophthalmol,* 2014:943786.

[35] Ibid. Kawashima. (2018).

[36] Feng, J, Chen, X, Sun, X, Wang, F, Sun, X. (2014). Expression of endoplasmic reticulum stress markers GRP78 and CHOP induced by oxidative stress in blue light-mediated damage of A2E-containing retinal pigment epithelium cells. *Ophthalmic Res,* 52(4):224-33.

[37] Tosini, G, Ferguson, I, Tsubota, K. (2016). Effects of blue light on the circadian system and eye physiology. *Mol Vis,* PMC4734149.

[38] Kruse, J. (2012). EMF 1: Does Your Rolex Work? Retrieved Nov 28 2017 from www.jackkruse.com/emf-1.

[39] Talwadkar, S., Jagannathan, A., Raghuram, N. (2014). Effect of trataka on cognitive functions in the elderly. *Int J Yoga*, Jul-Dec;7(2):96-103.

[40] Sabal, B.A., Wang, J., Cardenas-Morales, L., Faiq, M., Heim, C. (2018). Mental stress as consequence and cause of vision loss: the dawn of psychosomatic ophthalmology for preventative and personalized medicine. *EPMA J*, May 9;9(2):133-160.

[41] Cahn, B. R., Goodman, M.S., Peterson, C.T., Maturi, R., Mills, P.J. (2017). Yoga, Meditation and Mind-Body Health: Increased BDNF, Cortisol Awakening Response, and Altered Inflammatory Marker Expression after a 3-Month Yoga and Meditation Retreat. *Front Hum Neurosci*, 2017:11:315.

[42] Angelina, J. How Meditation Practices Help in Improving Eyesight. Retrieved Jul 9 2018 from https://www.mindbodygreen.com/0-15506/how-to-choose-the-right-meditation-technique-for-you.html.

[43] Williams, W. (2014). How to Choose the Right Meditation Technique for You. Retrieved Jul 9 2018 from https://www.mindbodygreen.com/0-15506/how-to-choose-the-right-meditation-technique-for-you.html

[44] Ibid. Talwadkar. (2014).

[45] Ibid. Williams. (2014).

[46] Ibid. Williams. (2014).

[47] T.F. Ross (2015). The Death of Textbooks? The Atlantic, Mar 6.

[48] Shantakumari, N., Eldeeb, R., Sreedharan, J., Gopal, K. (2014). Computer Use and Vision-Related Problems Among University Students In Ajman, United Arab Emirate. *Med Health Sci Res*,.4 Mar-Apr; 4(2): 258–263.

[49] Tatemichi M, Nakano T, Tanaka K, Hayashi, T., Nawa, T. et al. (2004). Possible association between heavy computer users and glaucomatous visual field abnormalities: a cross sectional study in Japanese workers. *J Epidemiol Community Health*, Dec;58(12):1021-7.

[50] Nakano, T., Hayaski, T., Nakagawa, T., Honda, T., Owada, S., et al. (2017). Increased Incidence of Visual Field Abnormalities as Determined by Frequency Doubling Technology Perimetry in High Computer Users Among Japanese Workers: A Retrospective Cohort Study. *J Epidemiol*, Nov 25.

[51] Uchino, Y., Uchino, M., Yokoi, N. (2014). Alteration of Tear Mucin 5AC in Office Workers Using Visual Display Terminals: The Osaka Study. *JAMA Ophthalmol*,132(8):985-992.

[52] Hunter, J.J., Morgan, J.I., Merigan, W.H., Sliney, D.H., Sparrow, J.R., et al. (2012). The susceptibility of the retina to photochemical damage from visible light. *Prog Ret Eye Res*, Jan;31(1):28-42.

[53] Narimatsu, Tl, Negishi, K., Miyake, S., Hirasawa, M., Osada, H., et al. (2015). Blue light-induced inflammatory marker expression in the retinal pigment epithelium-choroid of mice and the protective effect of a yellow intraocular lens material in vivo. *Exp Eye Res*, Mar;132:48-51.

[54] Logan, P., Bernabeu, M., Ferreira, A., Burner, M.N. (2015). Evidence for the Role of Blue Light in the Development of Uveal Melanoma. *J Ophthalmol*, 2015:386986.

[55] Charpe, N.A., Kaushik, V. (2009). Computer vision syndrome (CVS): Recognition and control in software professionals. *J Hum Ecol*, 2009;28:67–9

[56] Wimalasundera S. (2009). Computer vision syndrome. *Galle Med J*, 11(1):25–9.

[57] Fernandez-Montero, A., Olmo-Jimenez, J.M., Olmo, N., Bes-Rastroll, M., Moreno-Galarraga, L. , et al. (2015). The impact of computer use in myopia progression: a cohert study in Spain. *Prev Med*, Feb;71:67-71.

[58] Ibid. Tatemichi. (2004)..

[59] Abdelaziz, M.M., Fahim, S.A., Mousa, D.B., Gaya, B.I. (2009). Effects of computer use on visual acuity and colour vision. *Eur J Sci Res,* 2009;35:99–105.

[60] Bergqvist, U.O., Knave, B.G. (1994). Eye discomfort and work with visual display terminals. *Scand J Work Environ Health*, Feb; 20(1):27-33.

[61] Hitoe, S., Tanaka, J., Shimoda, H. (2014). MaquiBright™ standardized maqui berry extract significantly increases tear fluid production and ameliorates dry eye-related symptoms in a clinical pilot trial. *Panminerva Med,* Sep;56(3 Supple 1):1-6.

[62] Yamashita, S.I., Suzuki, N., Yamamoto, K., Iio, S.I., Yamada, T. (2018). Effects of MaquiBright on Improving Eye Dryness and Fatigue in Humans: A Randomized, Double-Blind, Placebo-Controlled Trial. *J Tradit Complement Med.* Nov 22;9(3):172-178.

[63] Kwon, J., Surenkhuu, I., Atassi, N., Mun, J., Chen, Y.F., et al. (2020). Pathological Consequences of Anti-Citrullinated Protein Antibodies in Tear Fluid and Therapeutic Potential of Pooled Human Immune Globulin-Eye Drops in Dry Eye Disease. *Ocul Surf. Jan;18(1):80-97.*

[64] Mun, C., Gulati S., Tibrewal, S., Chen, Y.F., An, S., et al. (2019). A Phase I/II Placebo-Controlled Randomized Pilot Clinical Trial of Recombinant Deosyribonuclease (DNase) Eye Drops Use in Patients with Dry Eye Disease. *Trans Vis Sci Tech.* 2019:8(3):10.

Other Books by Safe Goods

Natural Eye Care Series: Macular Degeneration	*$ 14.95*
Natural Eye Care Series: Glaucoma	*$ 14.95*
Natural Eye Care Series: Cataracts	*$ 14.95*
The Shattered Oak	*$ 14.95*
A Barnstormer Aviator	*$ 12.95*
Flying Above the Glass Ceiling	*$ 14.95*
Spirit & Creator (Spirit of St. Louis)	*$ 29.95*
Letters from My Son	*$ 22.95*
Nutritional Leverage for Great Golf	*$ 9.95*
Overcoming Senior Moments Expanded	*$ 9.95*
Prevent Cancer, Strokes, Heart Attacks	*$ 11.95*
Cancer Disarmed Expanded	*$ 7.95*
Eye Care Naturally	*$ 8.95*
Velvet Antler	*$ 9.95*

www.SafeGoodsPublishing.com